Authors

Samer S. Hoz, M.D., FABNS, FRCS (NeuroSurgery-Glasgow)
Department of Neurosurgery, Neurosurgery Teaching
Hospital, Baghdad, Iraq. Hozsamer2055@gmail.com

Zahraa F. Al-Sharshahi, M.D.
Department of Neurosurgery, Neurosurgery Teaching
Hospital, Baghdad, Iraq. zahraaalsharshahi@rcsi.com

Teeba M. Ghanim
Medical student interested in neurosurgery, College
of Medicine, University of Baghdad, Baghdad, Iraq.
teebamohammed12@yahoo.com

Ali M. Neamah
Medical student interested in neurosurgery, College of
Medicine, University of Baghdad, Baghdad, Iraq.
Ali.moh.neamah@gmail.com

Rasha Alaa Alshakarchy, M.D.
Department of Neurosurgery, Neurosurgery Teaching
Hospital, Baghdad, Iraq. ralaa16@gmail.com

Mustafa M. Altaweel, M.D.
Department of Neurosurgery, Neurosurgery Teaching
Hospital, Baghdad, Iraq. Mostafa_moh_h@yahoo.com

Alaa W. Arkawazi, M.D.
Department of Neurosurgery, Neurosurgery Teaching
Hospital, Baghdad, Iraq.
Alaawaly89@gmail.com.

Mustafa k. Ahmed
Medical student intrested in neurosurgery, kirkuk medical
college, Kirkuk, Iraq.
Mustafakhalidm14@gmail.com

Aktham O. Al-Khafaji
Medical student interested in neurosurgery, College of
Medicine, University of Baghdad, Baghdad, Iraq.
akthamalkhafaji@gmail.com

Mohammed A Al-Dhahir MD, IFAANS
Department of Neurosurgery, Strong Memorial Hospital,
601 Elmwood Ave, Rochester-NY 14642, New York-United
States.
dr.mohammed.aldhahir@gmail.com

Awfa A. Aktham
Department of Neurosurgery. Neurosurgery Teaching
Hospital, Baghdad, Iraq.
awfa.aktham@gmail.com

Zumurud A. mohammed
Department of Neurosurgery. Neurosurgery Teaching
Hospital, Baghdad, Iraq.
mohammdsalam@yahoo.com

Foreword One

If there was a prophecy about Neurosurgery in the recent times, I am certain it would speak volumes about the work that is being done out of Baghdad, by Samer and his colleagues. They have infused fresh life to an ailing Neurosurgery Which was bereft of skill and imagination.... and continues to inspire. The sketches, the quotes and the puzzles could be compared to a beautiful landscape complete with mountains, jungles and flowing rivers.... and that is where One longs to go, when tired...My best for the authors and I look forward to their further contributions

Iype Cherian
Neurosurgeon, Department of
Neurosurgery, COMS, Bharatpur, Nepal
Executive committee of the Asian association of neurosurgery.
Anatomy committee of the WFNS
(World Federation of Neurosurgery).

Foreword Two

The one who sees the future. 9 letters. Vertical.
Solution: VISIONARY

To understand this book the reader needs to focus on two aspects:

1. The definitions of "visionary" and "early innovator"
2. The mind behind this book
   - Being visionary means not only knowing the area to innovate, but also understanding how people in this area communicate and learn in the present and how all these things will evolve in the future. And not only. Most of all, it means going beyond what is considered as a standard. A visionary understands an important point: everything that is considered standard today was an innovation yesterday. Then, the visionary pushes himself into the dark, following a vision in mind, shedding light and paving the way for those who come next, and in the end, he suggests a new standard. This takes courage, because many innovations can be met with criticism at the start. But together with the visionary, we always find a group of early innovators, the first to understand and apply the news to guide the rest of the world in that revolution.

     Dr Samer Hoz is brave; he is a real visionary. You, reader, are an early innovator. This book is about this magic.
   - I met Dr. Samer Hoz 4 years ago. He introduced me to advancement in communication between

specialists that was taking place at the time: the birth of neurosurgery discussion groups on social media and instant messaging apps. Also, on that occasion, he was among the early innovators. From there, I discovered all the educational initiatives Dr. Hoz was carrying out with big determination. Just to mention a few, he founded the Hoz Neurosurgery Simulation Laboratory at the Neurosurgery Teaching Hospital of Baghdad, a place where innovative training is the basis for students and residents to explore the passion for neurosurgery. He coordinates the Continuing Medical Education program in the same department. He is a director of the Neurosurgical Research of the Iraqi Association of Neurological Surgeons. He is also a director and founder of the Neurosurgery Medical Student Elective Program in Iraq. As an early innovator, he was one of the first to understand what I was starting to do in 2016. In that period, I was working with my team on mobile-based systems for cranial approaches simulations. It was a first attempt, still immature, difficult to understand for the scientific community. But, once again, the innovator courageously showed interest in something absolutely new and non-standard. So, Dr. Hoz and his team published the first case report on the subject.

In this book, Dr. Hoz and his team explored a new frontier: cognitive learning applied to neuroscience. Thanks to their ability to involve young medical students and residents, giving them motivation and confidence in the future, they did this unique cognitive experiment to provide a disruptive method of mental training. This work is a delightful fusion between useful and enjoyable, between play and science. Using the deep connection between memory and emotion, they conceived an experimental method of memorization through the fun provided by gaming.

The effectiveness of this work will clarify to the reader the importance of being innovative even in the most repetitive things, such as the study of neurosciences.

This book suggests something even more important than the knowledge itself: the deep love for it.

Federico Nicolosi, MD
Consultant Neurosurgeon, Department of neurosurgery,
Humanitas Research Hospital, Milan. Italy
Founder and CEO of UpSurgeOn
Member of WFNS – Young Neurosurgeons Committee

Preface

The origin of crosswords can be traced back to the 19th century, England. It was not, however, until December 21, 1913, when the first crossword was published. The journalist, Arthur Wynne from Liverpool, is generally accredited with the invention of the game. Since its first appearance in the *New York World*, the game has conquered the world and created a craze in the field of entertainment. Crosswords puzzles dance on the wit of the human brain and who is a better performer than the brain surgeons themselves!

Neurosurgery is an intrinsically puzzling specialty that has been linked to creativity and innovation since its inception, so some more puzzles should do no harm! It is, at the same time, one of the most intellectually demanding, intensely stressful professions where mistakes are unacceptable, and failure is not an option. After a hectic day of long, intensive surgeries, the time comes to properly unwind and mentally prepare for what lies ahead. Caring for their fascination with science, we crafted this book to serve as a useful distractor for neurosurgeons during their well-deserved break time!

We are proud to introduce *The Neurosurgery Board Favorites: Crossword Puzzles* as the first of its kind, not only in neurosurgery but in all medical specialities. The intension of bringing out *this book* is to unravel the "lighter side" of learning neurosurgery if one truly exists! It is aimed as an entertaining refresher for neurosurgeons, neurosurgery residents, and medical students, alike. The book could well serve as a quiz question bank for the wards, but also as the stepping step for an upcoming series of more involved neurosurgery puzzle books. We hope that you find this book both interesting and useful.

Authors

About this Book

- *THE NEUROSURGERY BOARD FAVORITES: CROSSWORD PUZZLES* is the *FIRST PUZZLE BOOK* in the medical specialties dedicated to bring out the "lighter" aspect of studying neurosurgery.
- 50 *NEUROSURGERY-ORIENTED CROSS-WORD PUZZLES* with a total of *524 QUESTIONS* included. the puzzles arranged by topic and difficulty as "basic" and "advanced".
- Coverage includes general essential areas in neurosurgery, with a special focus on hard-to-retain facts.
- *COGNITIVE LEARNING APPLIED TO NEU-ROSCIENCE* is the premise of this book.
- *THE NEUROSURGERY BOARD FAVORITES: CROSSWORD PUZZLES* is thoroughly revised and designed by neurosurgeons for the neurosurgeons.
- *SURREALISM DRAWINGS AND INSPIRA-TIONAL QUOTES* spread throughout the book for short mind-stimulating breaks. (All drawings are courtesy of Teeba M. Ghanim)
- Answers for all puzzles are provided at the end of the book.
- *THE NEUROSURGERY BOARD FAVORITES: CROSSWORD PUZZLES* is intended as an entertaining refresher for neurosurgeons, neurosurgery trainees, and medical students.

Using this Book

1. The puzzles are of two levels of difficulty: basic (first 40 puzzles), and advanced (last 10 puzzles), with a total of 524 clues.
2. Each grid revolves around a neurosurgery-related theme! Keep that in mind when solving the puzzles!
3. Letters should be used to fill the grey-shaded squares (basic) or the white squares (advanced)
4. If you are not familiar with crossword puzzles, don't worry — it's very easy! The aim is to use the clues to find the words you need to fill in the grid.
   - Clues can be either Horizontal or Vertical. In the example grid below, the clue for one Vertical is 'type of neuroimaging for vessels'; this means that you are looking for a word with nine letters which will fit vertically in the grid (the answer is "angiography" by the way).
   - Where the word symbol (A) is present in the clue, meaning "ABBREVIATION", you should use the known abbreviation to substitute for the word. For example, the clue to the second horizontal line in "advanced" puzzle grid below is "Type of stroke that lasts less than 24 hours" (ABBREVIATION), which means that you have to find an abbreviation with three letters to fit horizontally in the grid, (TIA is the answer). (Note: Only internationally acknowledged medical abbreviations have been used).
   - Where the symbol (D) is found in the clue, meaning "distributed", you can fill the squares with letters of the word in any order.

- When the clue contains the symbol (O), meaning "opposite", the letters of the answer word should be arranged in reverse, i.e., right-to-left (horizontal) or bottom-to-top (vertical).
- Where the word "two thirds" appears next to the clue, only 2/3rd of the letters of the answer word should be used.
- Below are two examples of the "basic" and "advanced" puzzles, with the different types of clues explained above.

5. If you get stuck, our collection of surrealism art and inspirational quotes are there to help you recover!
6. Solutions of all the puzzles are provided at the end of the book! Although, we trust that you will give it a second try before deciding to quit!
7. Do not stress! You are allowed to discuss with a friend or Google! (Yes! We do not call it cheating here!)
8. If, however, you feel like running the extra mile, you can consult the following resources (The Handbook of Neurosurgery, www.Radiopedia.com, www.upsurgeon. com, the American Association of Neurosurgery website).

Dedication

To Dr. Saad Al-Witri and all Iraqi neurosurgeons, the warriors in white armours and scalpel swords, who are fighting difficulties and working with scarce resources. To our patients who are our source of inspiration and the ultimate aim behind all our efforts.

Contents

Section Three: Answers

Simplified Examples

Basic:

Horizontal	Vertical
2. Type of neuroimaging of choice for soft tissue.	1. Type of neuroimaging for vessels.

Answer:

	A	
	N	
	G	
	I	
	O	
	G	
M	R	I
	A	
	P	
	H	
	Y	

Advanced:

Neurosurgery	1	2	3	4	5	6	7	8	9	10
1	C	C								
2	T	I	A							
3		A	R	U	A					
4			E							
5			A							
6										
7										
8										
9										
10										

Horizontal	Vertical
1. Similar letters. 2. Type of stroke That lasts less than 24 hours (A). 3. Occur before seizure (O).	1. Type of neuroimaging used in trauma (A). 2. The main artery in anterior circulation (A) (D). 3. Territory.

Section One

Basic Level Neurosurgery
Crossword Puzzles

Puzzles 1-40

1. Facial nerve branches

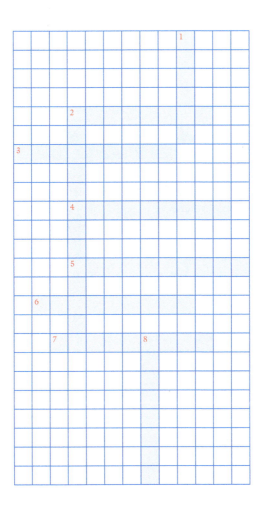

Horizontal	Vertical
2. Supplies platysma muscle.	1. Supplies buccinator muscle.
3. Supplies orbicularis oculi muscle.	2. Supplies taste sensation from the anterior 2/3 of the tongue.
4. Supplies auricularis posterior muscle.	8. Supplies frontalis muscle.
5. Supplies depressor labii inferioris muscle.	
6. Supplies stapedius muscle.	
7. Supplies the posterior belly of digastric and stylohyoid muscles.	

2. Areas without Blood Brain Barrier

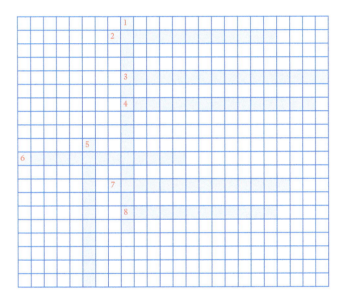

Horizontal	Vertical
2. Located in the hypothalamus between the optic chiasm and mammillary bodies and opened during Endoscopic Third Ventriculostomy .	1. Located on the under surface of the fornix near the foramen of Monro.
3. Related to lamina terminalis within the optic recess.	5. Part of the epithalamus called "the third eye" and responsible for melatonin production.
4. Stores and releases oxytocin and vasopressin.	
6. Responsible for the CSF production.	
7. Related to the optic chiasm and contains heat-sensitive neurons.	
8. Located in the lower part of the 4th ventricle floor and responsible for detection of circulating hormones involved in vomiting.	

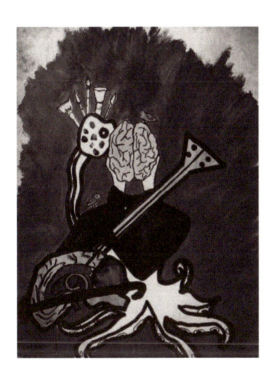

"The brain is wider
than the sky...."

Emily Dickinson

3. Intracranial Aneurysms

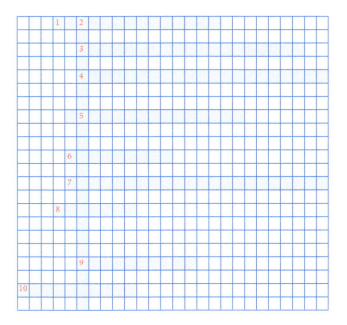

Horizontal	Vertical
1. The most common aneurysm to present with intracerebral hematoma.	2. Common in multiple aneurysms and is usually operated on through the anterior interhemispheric approach.
3. An aneurysm that mimics a pituitary mass when it is of large size.	
4. The most common intracranial aneurysm with male predominance.	
5. The most common site for giant aneurysms.	
6. Occurs after head injury and also called pseudoaneurysm.	
7. Usually presents with third nerve palsy.	
8. Most commonly caused by streptococcus viridans and Staphylococcus aureus.	
9. Accounts for 50 % of posterior circulation aneurysms.	
10. Total blindness is one of the sequelae for aneurysms of this type.	

4. Subarachnoid cisterns

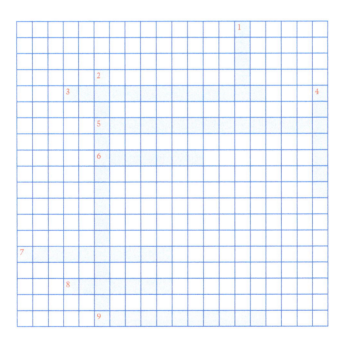

Horizontal	Vertical
3. Located posterior to the midbrain colliculi.	1. The largest cistern that is located behind medulla oblongata.
5. Contains the apex of the basilar artery.	2. Contains the anterior communicating artery complex.
6. Located between the quadrigeminal and crural cistern.	4. Contains the proximal part of the supraclinoid internal carotid artery.
7. Usually opened through endoscopic third ventriculostomy.	
8. Contains the middle cerebral artery.	
9. Located between the third ventricle and the sella turcica.	

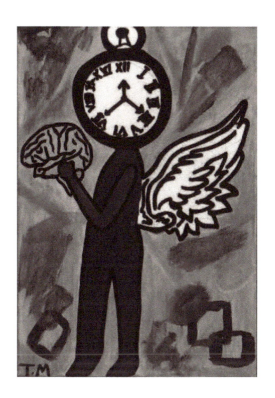

**"One must work with time
and not against it"**

Ursula K. Le Guin

5. Internal carotid artery branches

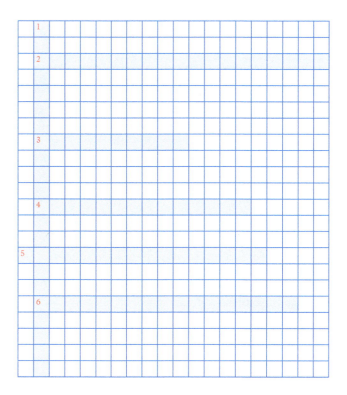

Horizontal	Vertical
2. Supplies the infundibulum and the pituitary gland.	1. Has an intimate relationship with the oculomotor nerve.
3. Supplies the orbit.	
4. The direct continuation of the internal carotid artery and has four segments.	
5. Related to the corpus callosum and has five segments.	
6. Its occlusion causes contralateral hemiparesis, hemi-anesthesia and hemianopia.	

6. External carotid artery branches

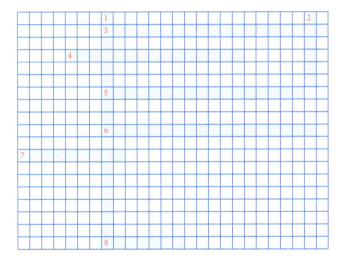

Horizontal	Vertical
3. Common donner site for extracranial-intracranial bypass.	1. The smallest branch of the external carotid artery and reaches the foramen lacerum.
4. The first branch of the external carotid artery.	2. Runs around the mandible and ends near the eye.
5. Runs in the infratemporal fossa and gives 17 branches.	
6. Originates above the posterior belly of the digastric and gives stylomastoid branch to the middle ear.	
7. Originates opposite to the facial artery and runs in a groove medial to the mastoid process.	
8. supplies the tongue.	

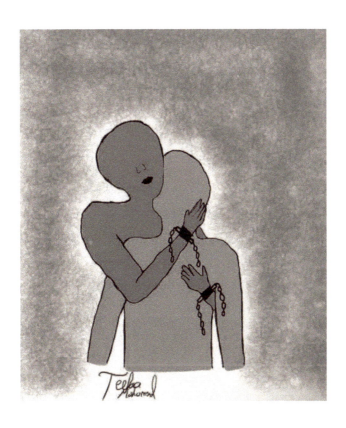

"You always gain
by giving love."

Reese Witherspoon

7. Persistent Carotid-vertebro-basilar anastomoses

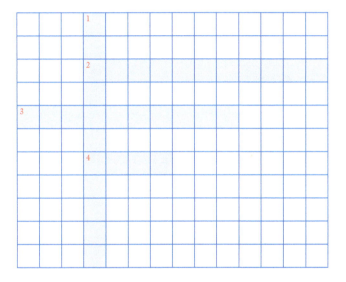

Horizontal	Vertical
2. Arises from the internal carotid artery and joins the vertebral CERVICAL artery at the V3 segment. 3. The most common variant that connects the cavernous to the internal carotid and basilar arteries. 4. Runs through the internal auditory canal to connect the petrous internal carotid artery to the proximal part of the basilar artery.	1. Arises from the extracranial part of the internal carotid artery and can cause glossopharyngeal nerve neuralgia.

8. Cerebral veins

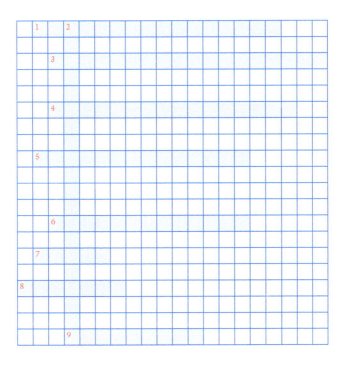

Horizontal	Vertical
1. Found in the superior part of the cerebellopontine space, also known as "vein of Dandy".	2. A vein that can be sacrificed during the supracerebellar infratentorial approach to the pineal region.
3. Runs in the Sylvian fissure and drains into the basal vein of Rosenthal.	
4. Runs in the velum interpositum inferiorly.	
5. Joins the septal vein to form the internal cerebral vein at the foramen of Monro.	
6. lies in the quadrigeminal cistern and unites with the inferior sagittal sinus to form the straight sinus.	
7. Connects the superficial middle cerebral vein to the transverse sinus.	
8. Anastomoses with the superficial middle cerebral vein and the superior sagittal sinus.	
9. Has an intimate relationship with the posterior cerebral artery and ends in the vein of Galen.	

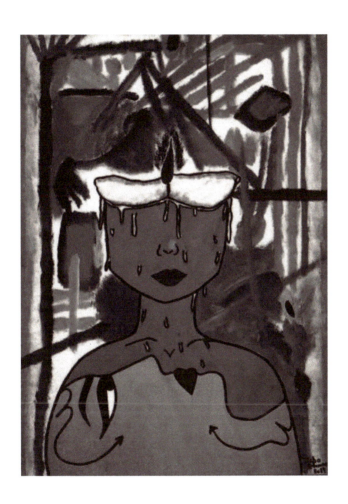

"There is no force so powerful as an idea whose time has come."

Everett Dirksen

9. Aphasias

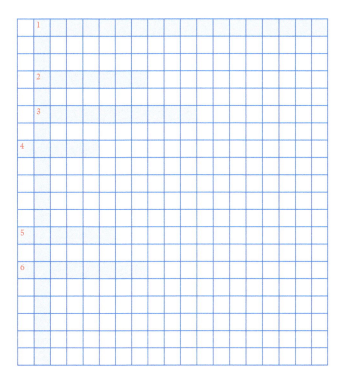

Horizontal	Vertical
1. Patient can't say a sentence but can repeat it.	1. Caused by tumors in the parieto- temporo-occipital junction area.
2. Characterized by fluent speech and complicated by word-finding difficulties.	
3. Caused by a damage to the arcuate fasciculus.	
4. Caused by an injury to broadmann area 44.	
5. The most severe of all subtypes of aphasia.	
6. Caused by an injury to the inferior temporal branch of the MCA.	

10. Craniometric points

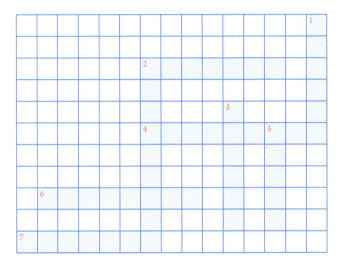

Horizontal	Vertical
2. Located on the sagittal suture at the level of parietal foramina.	1. Located at the central point of the parietal eminence.
4. Located between the coronal suture and the superior temporal line.	2. Identifies the level of the cervico-medullary junction.
6. Confluence point of the lambdoid, parietomastoid and occipitomastoid sutures.	3. Corresponds to the anterior margin of the foramen magnum at midline.
7. Corresponds to the area where the sphenoid wing articulates with the parietal, frontal and squamous part of the temporal bone.	5. Corresponds to the external occipital protuberance.

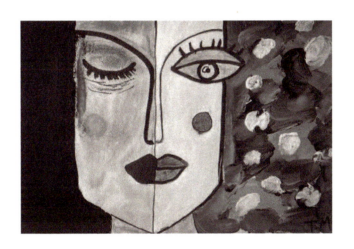

"The sun sees your body; the moon sees your soul"

Ankita Paul

11. Insertion points for ventriculo-peritoneal shunts

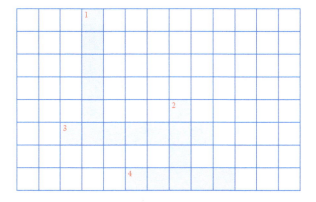

Horizontal	Vertical
3. Gives entry to the occipital horn of the lateral ventricle at 4cm from midline, 6cm above inion.	1. An entry point to the frontal horn of the lateral ventricle.
4. Gives entry to the occipital horn of the lateral ventricle at 2cm from midline, 3cm above inion.	2. An entry point to the atrium of the lateral ventricle.

12. The age of intracerebral hemorrhage based on MR imaging.

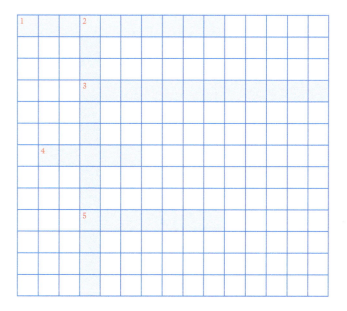

Horizontal	Vertical
1. Hematoma appears isointense on T1 and hyperintense on T2.	2. Hematoma appears after (3 to 7) days on MRI.
3. Hematoma appears bright on both T1 and T2.	
4. T2 signal intensity drops ((very hypointense)) in this hematoma.	
5. Hematoma appears hypointense on both T1 and T2.	

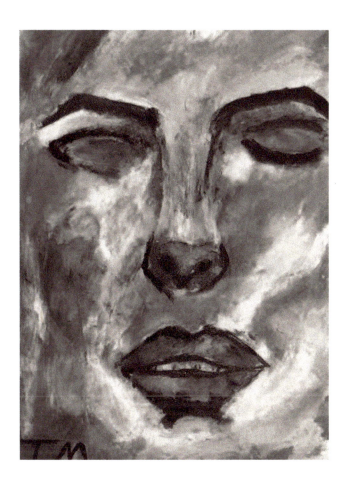

**"The future belongs
to those who believe
in the beauty of
their dreams"**

Eleanor Roosevelt

13. Cranial foramina

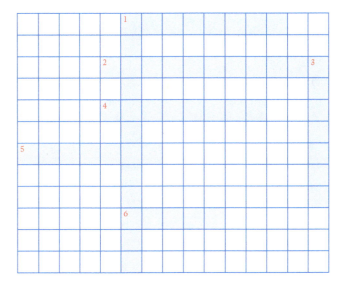

Horizontal	Vertical
1. Middle meningeal artery passes through it.	1. The extratemporal segment of the facial nerve passes through it.
2. Also called anterior condylar canal.	
4. Conveys the maxillary nerve.	3. Closed inferiorly with a membrane and the internal carotid artery exits from it to enter the cavernous sinus.
5. Conveys three cranial nerves with 70% of the parasympathetic fibers of the body passing through it.	
6. The motor fibers of the fifth cranial nerve pass through it.	

14. Arteries supplying the internal capsule

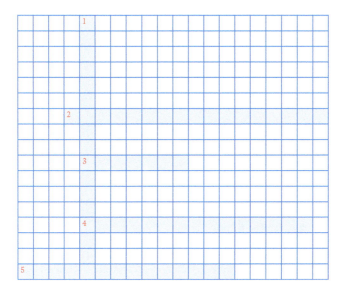

Horizontal	Vertical
2. Its striatal branches supply the retrolentiform and sublentiform parts of the internal capsule. 3. Supplies the lower part of the anterior limb and the genu. 4. Supplies the lower part of the posterior limb and the genu. 5. Supplies the upper part of the genu, anterior and posterior limbs.	1. Supplies the sublentiform and the lower part of the posterior limb.

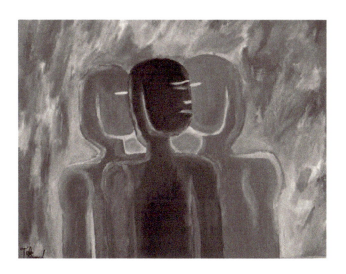

Self-power...

15. Brain herniation syndromes

Horizontal	Vertical
2. Characterized by compression of the posterior aspect of the midbrain with midsized fixed pupil and hyperventilation. 3. Characterized by ipsilateral fixed dilated pupil with or without contralateral hemiplegia. 4. Characterized by a downward displacement of the diencephalon 5. Also known as herniation through the foramen magnum.	1. Characterized by midline shift and may cause ACA infarction.

16. Differential diagnoses of intraparenchymal Ring enhancing lesions

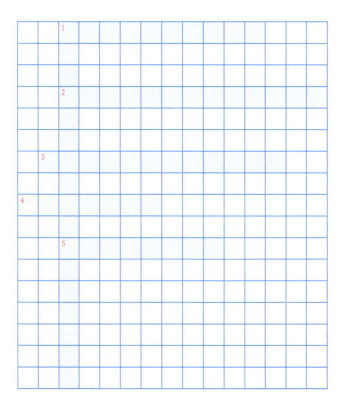

Horizontal	Vertical
1. The most common cause of multiple ring-enhancing lesions.	1. Characterized by an incomplete ring.
2. Commonly seen in HIV patients.	
3. The most common primary brain tumor causing ring enhancing lesions.	
4. Common in immunocompetent adult patient.	
5. Usually in immunocompromised patients.	

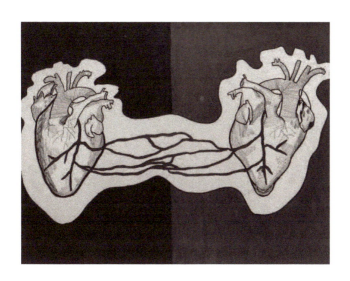

"Be your own soulmate!"

Solani Garg

17. Approaches to selective amygdalo-hippocampectomy

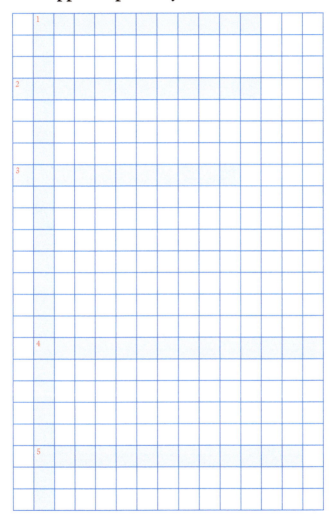

Horizontal	Vertical
1. Described by Park, 1996.	1. Described by Türe, 2012.
2. Described by Yasargil, 1982.	
3. Described by Rougier, 1992.	
4. Described by Vajkoczy, 1998.	
5. Described by Niemeyer, 1958.	

18. Types of lumbar interbody fusion

Horizontal	Vertical
3. Uses an oblique trajectory and gives access to L5-S1. 5. Indicated in patients with recurrent disc herniation and uses the bilateral posterolateral trajectory.	1. The most frequently used form of interbody fusion. 2. The best for restoration of lordosis and cannot access L1/2 and L2/3 because of the high risk of vascular injury. 4. Good option for the higher lumbar levels especially in deformity correction and cannot access L5-S1.

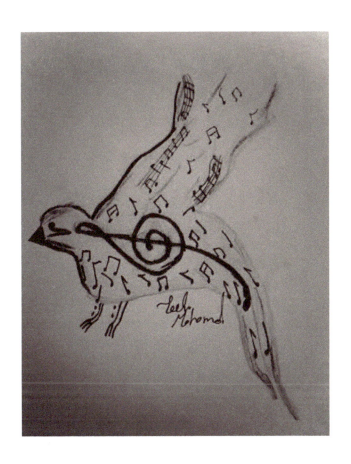

"Without music, life would be a mistake."

Friedrich Nietzsche

19. Types of craniosynostosis

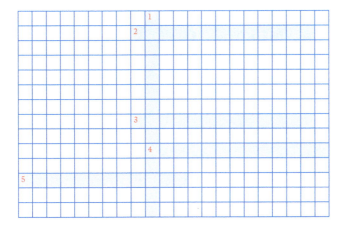

Horizontal	Vertical
2. Involves the bicoronal and/ or bilambdoid sutures.	1. Involves the metopic suture leading to a triangular forehead.
3. Involves the sagittal suture.	
4. Involves the unilateral coronal and lambdoid sutures.	
5. Involves the sagittal, coronal and lambdoid sutures (tower like skull).	

20. Phacomatosis

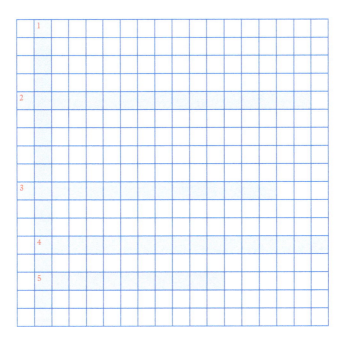

Horizontal	Vertical
2. Alternative name for type one Neurofibromatosis.	1. The most common phacomatosis.
3. A syndrome that consists of multiple Haemangioblastomas especially cerebellar.	
4. A syndrome that classically presents with adenoma sebaceum, seizure, and cortical tubers.	
5. A syndrome associated with facial hemangiomas and cortical calcifications.	

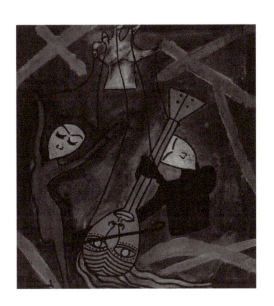

We fell for the idea of each other, but ideas are dangerous things to love!

21. Pineal region tumors

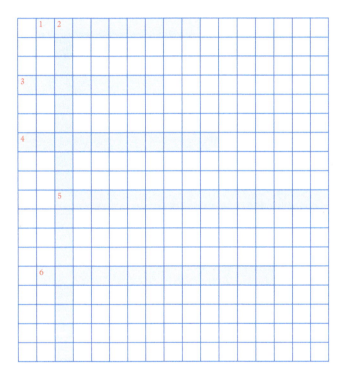

Horizontal	Vertical
1. The most common pineal tumor.	2. A malignant germ cell tumor with a propensity to metastasize systemically, associated with elevated Alpha-fetoprotein levels
3. Has hemorrhage in imaging and usually presents in infants.	
4. The most common benign pineal parenchymal tumor.	
5. A highly vascular and malignant tumor usually associated with elevated human chorionic gonadotropin levels.	
6. The most common malignant pineal parenchymal tumor usually presenting during the first and second decades of life.	

22. Peripheral nerves

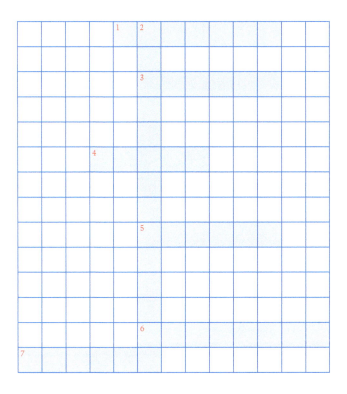

Horizontal	Vertical
1. Supplies the hamstrings muscles.	2. lesion of this nerve at the fibular neck causes foot drop with loss of eversion.
3. Affected in the most common peripheral nerve compression syndrome.	
4. The most common site for entrapment of this nerve is at the elbow (cubital tunnel syndrome)	
5. Lesion of this nerve causes wrist drop.	
6. Supplies the teres minor muscle.	
7. Supplies the sole of the foot.	

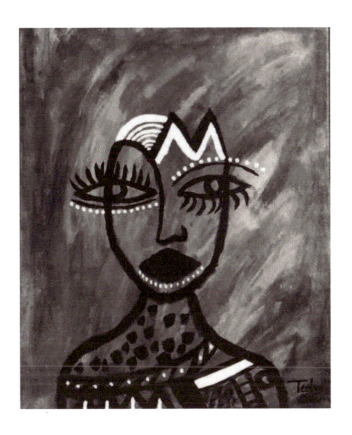

"It is weird not to be weird!"

John Lennon

23. Types of meningioma according to the location

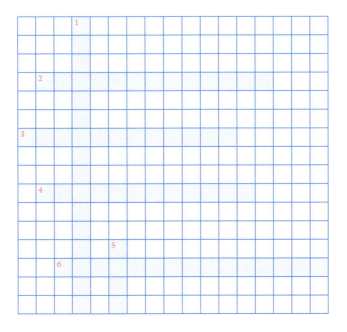

Horizontal	Vertical
2. Can present with rotatory paralysis of the four limbs.	1. Most frequently (up to **80%**) located at the trigone of the lateral ventricles and usually on the left side.
3. Divided into three groups, the medial one also termed as clinoidal meningioma.	5. Differentiated from parasagittal meningioma by being covered with brain tissue upon dural opening.
4. Its extension into the superior sagittal sinus is classified by Sindou grading system.	
6. Usually presents with cognitive impairment and behavioral changes.	

24. Histopathological types of meningioma

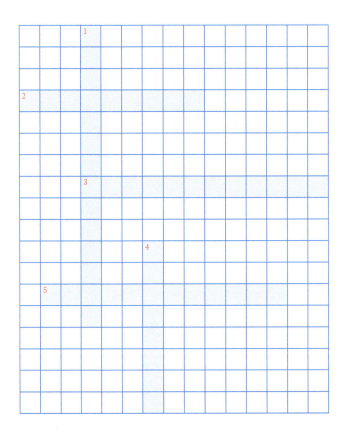

Horizontal	Vertical
2. Grade III WHO meningioma with its cells having elongated processes. 3. Has intermediate features between meningothelial and fibroblastic meningiomas. 5. Commonly found in the spine and characterized by numerous psammoma bodies.	1. The most common meningioma histology. 4. Grade II WHO meningioma and contains chordoid cells.

25. Cerebral metastasis

Horizontal	Vertical
2. Organ of origin for 1-2% of the brain metastasis.	1. Predominately cystic with a marginal enhancing solid component and can show hemorrhagic changes.
4. Has the highest tendency for brain metastasis.	
5. The most common source of brain metastasis.	3. Commonly metastasizes to the leptomeninges.
6. Usually presents with hemorrhagic metastasis and thyrotoxicosis.	
7. Commonly found in the posterior pituitary and the suprasellar region and may cause osteoblastic changes if it involves the bone.	

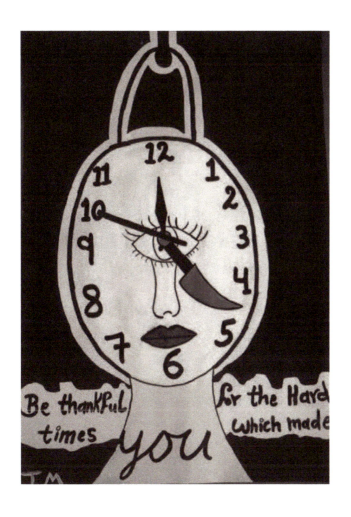

"Be thankful for the hard times, for they have made you"

Leonardo Wilhelm DiCaprio

26. Jugular foramen syndromes

Horizontal	Vertical
2. involvement of 10, 11 cranial nerves.	1. involvement of 10, 12 cranial nerves.
4. involvement of 9, 10, 11 cranial nerves, intracranial lesion.	3. involvement of 9, 10, 11, 12 cranial nerves, extra-cranial lesion.
5. involvement of 9, 10, 11, 12 cranial nerves plus sympathetic plexus, retropharyngeal lesion.	
6. involvement of 10, 11, 12 cranial nerves.	

27. CSF shunt complications

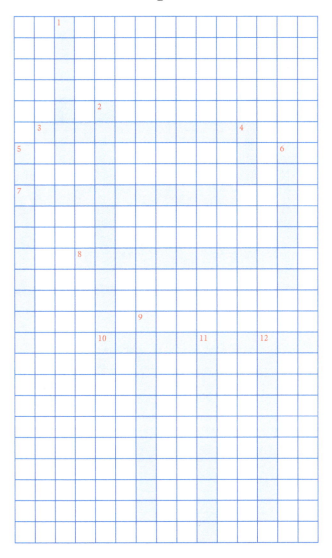

Horizontal	Vertical
3. transmission of intracranial infection to peritoneal cavity.	1. poor peritoneal CSF absorption.
7. occur during ventricular catheter placement	2. occur during growth of a child.
	4. occurs due to over-shunting.
peritoneal catheter migration inside bowel lumen.	5. Occurs due to poor haemostasis.
10. shunting a turbid CSF.	6. in association with intraventricular tumours.
	9. Occurs due to multiple peritoneal adhesions.
	11. Occurs due to thin skin and chronic pressure.
	12. Characterized by fever and elevated WBC.

28. Occipito-cervical junction ligaments

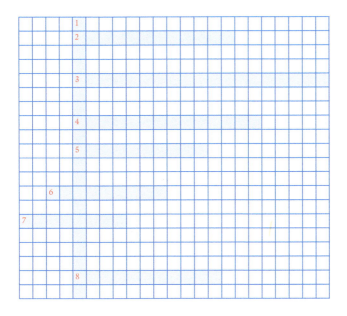

Horizontal	Vertical
2. connects dens to occipital condyle.	1. connects the posterior margin of foramen magnum to posterior arch of C1.
3. superior extension of anterior longitudinal ligament.	
4. Connects dens to basion.	
5. prevents posterior dislocation of dens.	
6. superior extension of posterior longitudinal ligament.	
7. joins C2, C1 and clivus.	
8. connects dens to lateral mass of C1.	

29. brainstem infarction syndromes

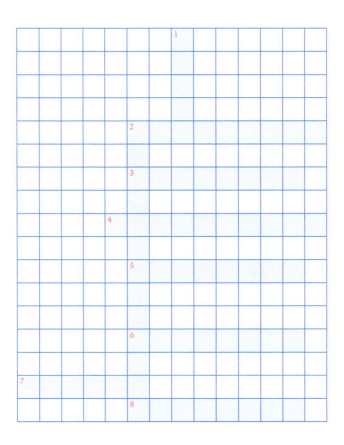

Horizontal	Vertical
2. ipsilateral CN VII, CN VIII, ataxia plus contralateral hemiplegia and hemianaesthesia.	1. ipsilateral CN III palsy plus contralateral hemiplegia.
3. conscious patient with paralysis of all voluntary muscles except those supplied by CN III.	2. ipsilateral CN VI + CN VII palsy plus contralateral hemiplegia.
4. ipsilateral facial sensory loss plus partial Horner plus bulbar muscle weakness plus vertigo and nystagmus plus contralateral hemianaesthesia.	
5. ipsilateral CN XII plus contralateral hemiplegia and hemianaesthesia.	
6. ipsilateral CN III palsy plus contralateral hemiplegia and ataxia.	
7. ipsilateral CN III palsy plus contralateral ataxia.	
8. mixed medial and lateral medullary findings.	

30. Spinal cord syndromes

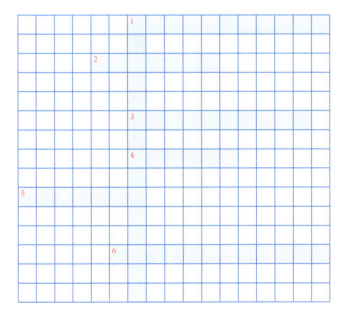

Horizontal	Vertical
1. presents with saddle anaesthesia plus only lower motor neuron deficit. 2. characterized by cape like sensory loss. 3. loss of all function below injured level. 4. loss of vibration and proprioception only. 5. due to anterior spinal artery occlusion. 6. also known as hemi cord syndrome.	1. presents with saddle anaesthesia plus urinary retention.

31. Nerve supply

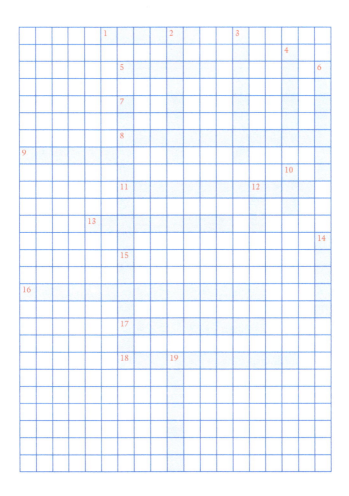

Horizontal	Vertical
1. soleus and gastrocnemius muscle.	2. deltoid muscle.
5. abductor pollicis brevis muscle.	3. external urethral sphincter muscles.
8. supraspinatus and infraspinatus muscles.	4. triceps muscle.
9. diaphragm muscle.	6. quadriceps femoris muscle.
11. serratus anterior muscle.	7. biceps brachii muscle.
13. trapezius muscle.	10. extensor digitorum muscle.
15. latissimus dorsi muscle.	12. flexor pollicis longus muscle.
16. gluteus maximus muscle.	14. interossei muscles.
17. adductor longus muscle.	19. biceps femoris muscle.
18. teres major muscle.	

32. Cerebral sulci

Horizontal	Vertical
3. Separate the cuneus from the precuneus.	1. Separate the frontal and temporal lobes, also called Sylvian fissure.
5. Separate the frontal and parietal lobes.	2. Surrounds the corpus callosum.
6. Located on lateral surface, inferior to Brodman area 8, and superior to The Broca's area.	4. Located between pars tringularis and pars opercularis, it is a ramus of lateral fissure.
7. Located in frontal lobe, between Brodman areas 4 and 6.	
8. The angular gyrus is wrapped around its posterior end.	
9. Surrounds the cingulum (cingulate gyrus).	
10. Divides the parietal lobe into superior and inferior parietal lobules.	
11. Separate the precuneus from the paracentral lobule.	
12. Located in the occipital lobe, connected to the parieto-occipital sulcus to form the Y shape sulcus on medial surface.	
13. Located in parietal lobe, between Brodman areas 3 and 5.	

33. Cerebral gyri - surface anatomy

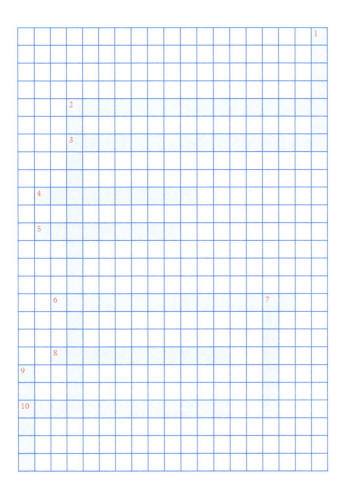

Horizontal	Vertical
2. Located In the temporal lobe, Contains the Wernicke's area in its posterior one third.	1. Wrapped around the posterior end of the superior temporal sulcus.
3. Represents Brodman area 45 and its function is motor of speech.	2. Represents Brodman area 6 and its function is initiation of the movement.
4. Represents Brodman area 4, its function is primary motor cortex.	
5. Located on medial surface. It is the continuation of the superior parietal lobule.	7. Located on medial surface in occipital lob, just anteromedial to calcarine sulcus, it's function is vision.
6. Represents Brodman area 8, its damage causes deficits in voluntary eye movement to the contralateral visual field.	
	9. Represents the primary auditory cortex.
8. Represents Brodman area 3,2,1 and its function is primary somatosensory cortex.	
10. Injury to it on dominant side causes Gertsman syndrome.	

34. Pupil abnormalities

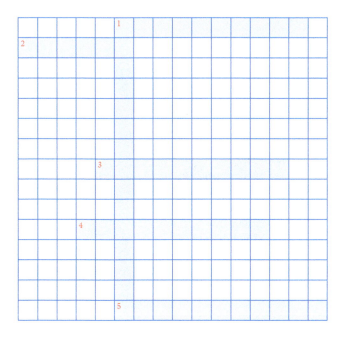

Horizontal	Vertical
1. asymmetrical pupil size.	1. irregular small pupil, caused by neurosyphilis.
2. Occurs in association with carotid dissection.	
3. also called tonic pupil, caused by degeneration of the ciliary ganglion.	
4. caused by relative afferent pupillary defect.	
5. Occurs due to complete CN III lesion	

35. Peripheral nerve palsy syndromes

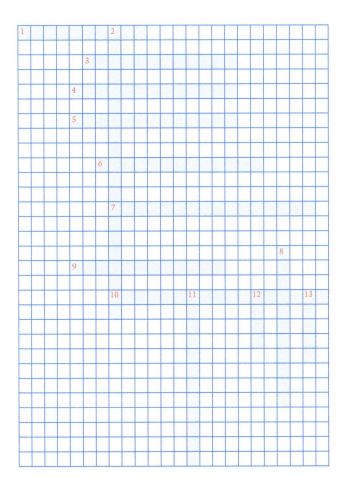

Horizontal	Vertical
1. sciatic nerve palsy due to compression by piriformis muscle.	2. occurs in tight belt users due to lateral femoral cutaneous nerve compression.
3. median nerve entrapment at the wrist.	
4. ascending inflammatory polyneuropathy.	8. ulnar nerve compression at the wrist.
5. ulnar nerve compression at the elbow.	11. tibial nerve entrapment at the ankle.
6. radial nerve palsy due to prolonged direct pressure on the upper medial arm.	12. due to brachial plexus injury.
7. peroneal nerve injury due to prolonged squatting.	13. delayed ulnar nerve compression.
9. peroneal nerve palsy due to prolonged sitting with crossed legs.	
10. hereditary polyneuropathy.	

36. The Orbit

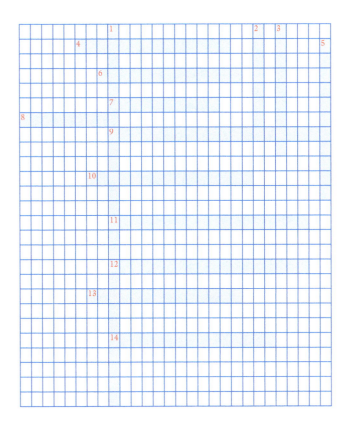

Horizontal	Vertical
4. One of the EOMs, function: depression of the eyeball.	1. One of the EOMs, function: elevation of the upper eyelid and maintain the upper eyelid position.
6. One of the EOMs, function: abduction of the eyeball.	
7. One of the CNs, pass through the annulus of Zinn, supply all of the EOMs except 2 of them.	
8. One of the CNs, pass through the superior orbital fissure, supply the superior oblique muscle.	2. One of the CNs, pass through the Dorello's canal, supply the lateral rectus muscle.
9. Also called iris sphincter muscle, supplied by the 3rd CN, function: constriction of the pupil.	3. Artery pass to orbit within the dura of the optic nerve.
10. One of the EOMs, function: internal rotation, abduction and depression of the eyeball.	5. One of the EOMs, function: adduction of the eyeball.
11. Artery pass through the superior orbital fissure.	
12. Vein communicates with the angular vein, it passes between the 2 heads of the lateral rectus, and through the superior orbital fissure.	
13. One of the EOMs, function: elevation of the eyeball.	
14. One of the EOMs, function: external rotation, abduction and elevation of the eyeball.	

37. Spinal cord tracts

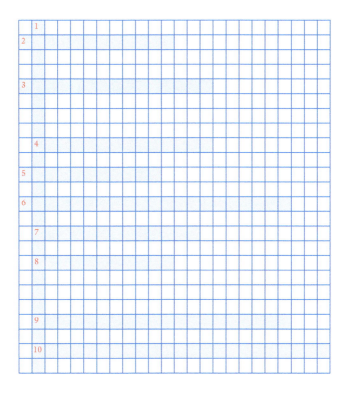

Horizontal	Vertical
2. Joint position, fine touch, vibration.	1. stretch reflex.
3. Facilitates extensor muscle tone.	
4. Automatic respiration.	
5. Nociceptive.	
6. Crude touch	
7. Skilled movement.	
8. Maintains flexor muscle tone.	
9. Pain and temperature.	
10. Whole limb position	

38. Magnetic Resonance Spectroscopy (MRS)

Horizontal	Vertical
1. Marker for membrane synthesis, cell marker.	1. Reference to choline, higher in gray than white mater.
2. Increased in necrotic tissue.	
3. Tallest peak in normal brain parenchyma.	

39. Complications of Subthalamic Nucleus (STN) Deep Brain Stimulation (DBS).

The following occur when the electrode is placed wrongly relative to the target nucleus

Horizontal	Vertical
2. miosis and diplopia. 3. Ataxia. 4. paresthesia. 5. flushing and sweating. 6. dysarthria.	1. tonic contraction.

40. Dermatomal levels

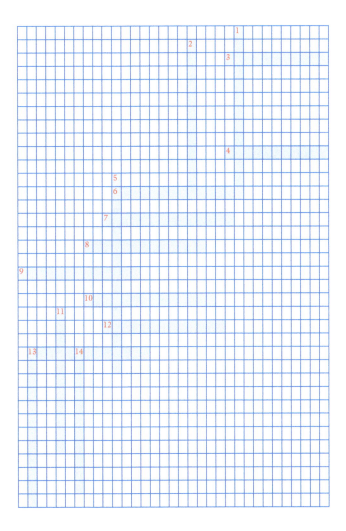

Horizontal	Vertical
3. inguinal ligament.	1. In the supraclavicular fossa, at the midclavicular line.
4. small toe.	
6. little finger.	
7. at least one cm lateral to the occipital protuberance at the base of the skull.	2. medial malleolus and Big toe medially.
8. thumb finger.	5. middle finger.
9. at umbilical level.	11. dorsum of foot & 3 middle toes.
10. at nipple level.	13. at the midpoint of the popliteal fossa.
12. lateral shoulder.	14. medial aspect of the knee joint.
13. xiphoid.	

Section Two

Advanced Level Neurosurgery
Crossword Puzzles

Puzzles 1-10

1. Pediatric neurosurgery

	1	2	3	4	5	6	7	8	9	10
1										
2										■
3			■			■				
4				■	■	■	■		■	■
5				■	■					■
6										
7			■							
8					■			■		
9		■			■					■
10										

Horizontal	Vertical
1. Fronto-ethmoidal encephalocele.	1. Early closure of cranial sutures (O).
2. Common complication of CSF shunt.	2. Part of vermis herniate in Chiari type 2.
3. 2/3 of CSF – similar letters – a possible content of dermoid cyst (D).	3. Neurocutaneous syndrome (A) - similar letters – preoperative order (O).
4. In the lower limb (D).	4. A tumor marker elevated in leptomeningeal spread of lung and breast CA – found in hydatid.
5. 3/4 Rare malignant pediatric tumor with a unique feature of central cystic area- 1/2 molecule (O).	5. Vessel involved in Moyamoya disease (A) – Hormone with pulsatile secretion, primarily at night (A) – muscle supplied by deep peroneal nerve (A).
6. A complication of untreated ruptured meningocele (O).	6. A lab test used to monitor Warfarin – related to genetics (O).
7. Similar letters- found in hepatitis.	7. Fenestration of the optic nerve is one of its treatment options (A) – herniate in Chiari type 1 (O).
8. Part of the ventricular system (O) – cranial nerve compression syndromes (A) – part of Cushing response (A).	8. The first part of craniosynostosis type denotes early closure of metopic suture (D) - related to genetics.
9. A lab test used to monitor Heparin - first part of craniosynostosis type denotes early closure of many or all sutures.	9. Antibody specific to nuclear antigens associated with SLE and antiphospholipid syndrome (A) - first part of drug not recommended any more for spinal cord injury based on the recent guidelines.
10. Associated with Alpert syndrome.	10. Parameter used in CT perfusion.

A: Abbreviated. D: Distributed. O: Opposite

2. Vascular neurosurgery (1)

	1	2	3	4	5	6	7	8	9	10
1										
2				■						
3				■	■					
4						■		■	■	
5						■				
6		■				■				
7					■				■	■
8										
9		■								
10					■		■			

Horizontal	Vertical
1. Type of vascular lesions of the brain that can present with tinnitus.	1. Should be opened during some cases of paraclinoid aneurysms clipping.
2. Unit used for detecting reversal of platelet inhibition in response to aspirin (A) (O) - famous study describing carotid endarterectomy (D).	2. Famous study related to cerebral AVM – can be associated with SAH.
3. Type of recording for deep brain activity (O) – part of "calvarium".	3. Type of vascular lesions with no arterial feeders nor venous drainage (D).
4. Famous British randomized controlled trial on the effect of Nimodipine in patients with subarachnoid hemorrhage (D).	4. A structure that represents a pathway for anterior circulation aneurysm surgery (D).
5. Type of AVM that can present with SAH in rare instances (O) – a serious post-operative complication.	5. A joint affected in ankylosing spondylitis (O) – thrombolytic agent (A).
6. Denotes motor neuron disease (O) – type of inflammatory response (A).	6. Artery used for EC-IC bypass surgery (A) – procedure used to treat Moyamoya disease (O).
7. A type of neck brace that extends from the sternum to the occiput (O) – brain stem structure related to wakefulness (O).	7. Recent large study of ruptured intracranial saccular aneurysms that showed no difference in clinical outcome between clipping and coiling (O) – A study describes the treatment of asymptomatic carotid atherosclerosis with endarterectomy (O).
8. The last structure to be closed during cerebral AVM resection (O) - endovascular embolization material (O).	8. Single – new type of operative room where both open and endovascular procedures can be done on the same patient on the same table (O).
9. Vascular disease of the brain that results in ischemia in children and hemorrhage in adults (O).	9. Part of "leukemia" – innovative technology included recently in neurosurgical training (A) – neuro-monitoring during the surgery (A) (O).
10. An ultrasonic wave-based device used for brain tumor resection (D) – a type of infection related to toxoplasmosis and lymphoma.	10. Type of cerebral revascularization (O) – found in "AVM".

A: Abbreviated. D: Distributed. O: Opposite

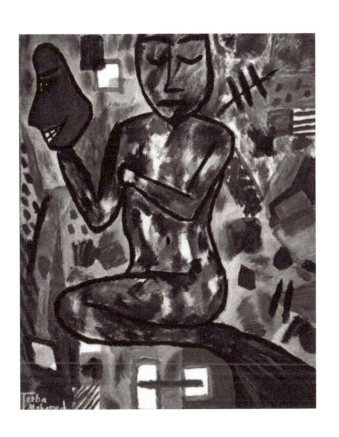

"We are what we pretend
to be, so we must be
careful about what we
pretend to be."

Kurt Vonnegut

3. Vascular neurosurgery (2)

	1	2	3	4	5	6	7	8	9	10
1									■	
2										
3				■				■		
4				■				■		
5				■				■		■
6				■						
7										
8	■			■			■			■
9				■		■		■		
10				■	■					

Horizontal:	Vertical:
1. Vascular malformation of the brain.	1. Common vascular malformation of the brain- can be associated with subarachnoid hemorrhage.
2. Type of results appear normal although they are abnormal upon testing (D).	2. An essential tool for deep brain stimulation.
3. Type of sensory fibers from the viscera conveyed by cranial nerves - ¾ of vascular tool – 2/3 of few.	3. Common presentation of AVM (O).
4. The correct name for pseudotumor cerebri – ¾ of important test before contrast administration (D)– not burst (A).	4. A risk factor for skin CA.
	5. Tumor appears again in the same site.
5. ½ of Proliferation (D)	6. Common presentation of AVM (O).
6. Found in upper limb (D)- 2/3 of one of the periventricular commissures.	7. Muscle supplied by anterior division of mandibular nerve(O).
7. Gene found to be associated with recurrent falls (D).	8. Used for histopathology (O)- vital sign decrease in Cushing's response.
8. Not a route for carbamazepine- endocrine syndrome (O).	9. Can present with pulsatile proptosis (O).
9. supplied by 3rd, 4th and 6th cranial nerves (O)- important cranial venous sinus (A).	10. Pathway of Everolimus- suicide neurosurgical disease (A)- (SIMILAR).
10. Used for TB treatment- seizure attack (D).	

4. Neuro-oncology

Horizontal:	Vertical:
1. A metastatic cancer with osteoblastic features (O).	1. A common intracranial tumor (O).
2. ½ injury (O)- rare malignant pediatric tumor (O).	2. A possible feature of meningioma in the geriatric population.
3. Found on the ventral surface of medulla oblongata- prominent sulcus between parietal and occipital lobe (A) (O).	3. Found in Intermediate.
	4. A type of CSF shunt (A)- found in remedy.
4. A common aneurysm (A)-one of the methods to treat trigeminal neuralgia (A) (O)- drug delivery route (O).	5. Immunohistochemical stain positive in meningioma, craniopharyngioma and pituitary adenoma (O)- first part of tumor that commonly shows calcification.
5. A body system that can rarely be a source of brain metastasis- found in Panadol.	6. first part of the syndrome of hemisection of the spinal cord.
6. A common phacomatosis syndrome (A) - Found in Emboliform.	7. A lesion that can contain teeth and hair (D).
7. Similar letters- found in Laterality.	8. Theater (A) – A feature CSF in traumatic tap (D).
8. Secreted from the adrenal gland (A) – grade 3 meningioma (O).	9. The commonest tumor in infant (D).
9. A tumor difficult to distinguish from normal parenchyma (O).	10. Grade 3 meningioma.
10. The commonest adult sellar mass (O).	

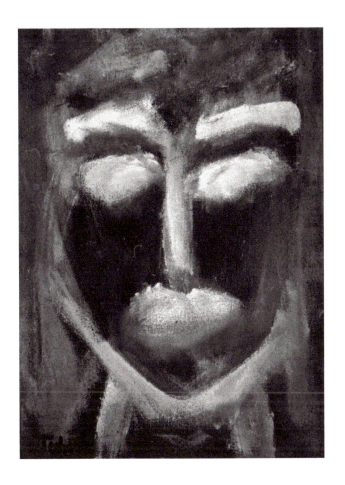

"You just have to trust your own madness!"

Clive Barker

5. Functional neurosurgery

	1	2	3	4	5	6	7	8	9	10
1										
2									■	
3										
4				■	■					
5		■					■			
6								■		
7	■		■				■			
8				■						
9									■	
10			■						■	■

Horizontal	Vertical
1. Off-label indication for VNS or DBS.	1. Neuronal pathway of Parkinson disease includes the GP interna – DBS target for refractory Parkinson (A).
2. Main indication for VNS (D).	
3. Found in "Galassi Grade".	2. Part of new device for endovascular treatment of aneurysm (O) – a possible content of dermal cyst (O).
4. A nucleus form part of indirect pathway of Parkinson disease but not used as a target for DBS (O) – found in "pannus" (D).	3. First part of craniosynostosis type denotes early closure of coronal or lambdoid suture – thyrotoxicosis (A) (O).
5. 2/3 of "Intact" (D) – recent imaging method for neuronal tract (A).	4. Found in "years" - signal transduction pathway used in medulloblastoma genetic classification (O) – vital sign decrease in Cushing response (O).
6. Found in "prolactinomas" (D) – marker for muscle injury (A).	
7. Hyponatremia with weight loss and dehydration (A) (O)- usual site of compression of trigeminal nerve in trigeminal neuralgia (A) (O).	5. Neurological investigation – famous trial studying carotid endarterectomy.
	6. Treated with intrathecal pump when medically refractory.
	7. Used for intraoperative monitoring – pathway for new drug targeting SEGA-
8. New treatment for medically refractory movement disorders (A) (O) – found in "carotid".	8. Used with Gigli saw for craniotomy (D) - part of anthelminthic drug.
9. Drug of choice for neuralgia.	9. One of the routes for urgent baclofen administration (O).
10. Part of midbrain rich in dopamine (A) (O) – found in "hydrate".	10. DBS is one of its treatment options (O).

A: Abbreviated. D: Distributed. O: Opposite

6. Neurotrauma

	1	2	3	4	5	6	7	8	9	10
1										
2										
3						■				■
4			■		■		■			
5									■	
6										
7				■		■				
8									■	
9									■	
10	■				■					

Horizontal	Vertical
1. Post-traumatic brief drop in neurological function with normal imaging.	1. Rare type of gunshot wound to the head when the bullet penetrates the skull then changes its direction and runs in the the subdural space without entering the brain parenchyma.
2. Found in aponeurosis.	
3. A ratio used for radiographic evaluation of atlanto-occipital dislocation (O) – suturing of the injured nerve ends with large stitch size during initial exposure when the lost nerve segment is too large for direct micro-anastomosis (O).	2. Surgeries (D).
	3. Recent – found in "indicator".
	4. A type of shunt device, also called Hakim or H-V valve (D) – more important for comatose patients than for neurological assessment (O).
4. Repeated seizures with no recovery between attacks (O) – 1/3 difficult.	5. Can be used to monitor post-traumatic pituitary dysfunction – used for feeding in the ICU (D).
5. An intracranial hematoma usually resulting from a coupe- type injury.	
6. Investigation required for post traumatic midline cervical tenderness (O).	6. Similar letters – acute phase reactant that is more sensitive than ESR as an indicator for infection (O) – found in "indo".
7. For imaging of neuronal tracts (O) - Procedure includes radical decompression of nerve roots with total facetectomy for spondylolisthesis (O).	7. Used for outcome assessment after TBI (O) - name of a retractor used in the transnasal approach (D).
	8. Found in "ill-microcephalus" (D).
8. Its rostral part involved in diffuse axonal injury (O).	9. Found in "outlet" – this means (O).
9. Type of skull fracture in young children (O).	10. Similar letters – a type of bullet injury to the head causing depressed fracture with no penetration to the parenchyma.
10. A prefix that indicates a tumor – small wound during perforating head injury by bullet.	

A: Abbreviated. D: Distributed. O: Opposite

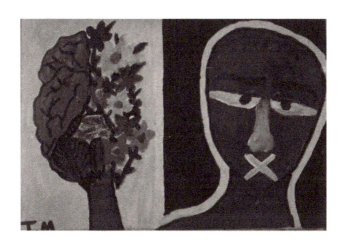

We all wear scars, they are
the source of light for us.

7. Spine

	1	2	3	4	5	6	7	8	9	10
1							■			
2					■					
3								■		■
4						■				
5	■	■					■			
6				■						
7							■			
8						■			■	
9					■					
10	■									■

Horizontal	Vertical
1. Yellow ligament of the spine – stands for Turcot syndrome (an autosomal dominant syndrome that includes colonic polyps and brain tumor).	1. A type of lateral interbody fusion of the spine with retroperitoneal exposure anterior to the psoas and lumbar plexus – common anterior approach to the cervical spine (A).
2. Radiation-induced optic neuropathy (D)- found in "lateral".	2. A force act on the spine – test for sacroiliac rather than lumbar spinal pathology (D).
3. Another name for straight-leg raising sign.	3. "Insular SBM" method (D).
4. Classification of degenerative changes of the spine based on MRI features (D)– expected complication of unintended durotomy (D).	4. Found in "Verbiest" syndrome – found in "phrenic".
5. A commonly used angle to assess the degree of scoliosis (O) – 3/4 "onyx".	5. Found in "costalgia".
6. Allergic fungal sinusitis that often involves bone destruction and extension into the orbit and anterior skull base (A) – found in "scallop".	6. Found in "Filum" – an institute provides leadership, best practices, research, support and training for a focus area (e.g.: neurosurgery) – found in "Gill".
7. A type of disc herniation causing myelopathy rather than radiculopathy (D) – related to blood.	7. Similar letters – related to spinal cord (D).
8. Portion of a facet joint that can be removed without affection of stability (O) - similar letters.	8. A type of infection that usually involves multiple adjacent vertebrae (O) – suffix denotes beta-blocking drugs – unstable atlanto-axial complex (A).
9. Post-laminectomy epidural fibrosis (A) (O) - special MRI image for cervical disc with the disc, CSF and flowing blood are of high signals.	9. Grading system for myelopathy (O) - similar letters.
10. A trochanteric lesion included in the differential diagnosis of neurological claudication.	10. A clinical test used in Coccydynia evaluation (A) – 3/4 of common sagittal spine pathology.

A: Abbreviated. D: Distributed. O: Opposite

8. Peripheral nerves

	1	2	3	4	5	6	7	8	9	10
1										
2		■								■
3							■			
4			■		■	■	■			
5							■		■	
6		■		■						
7					■	■		■		
8			■							
9		■		■	■					
10										

Horizontal	Vertical
1. Treatment option for occipital neuralgia.	1. Syndrome of tenosynovitis of the abductor pollicis longus and extensor pollicis brevis tendons included in the differential diagnosis of carpal tunnel syndrome (O).
2. Palsy of the lower brachial plexus (C8, T1) from traction of an abducted arm with characteristic claw deformity (D).	2. Direct continuation of popliteal artery that runs in the posterior compartment of the leg (A) - similar letters.
3. A clinical test for carpal tunnel syndrome (D) - when enters the skull, it's called intracranial aerocele or pneumocephalus (O).	3. Found in "skull"- a term used for thrombectomy of stroke denotes the time from patient's entry through the door of the ER to the needle insertion for catheterization (A) – radiological test (O).
4. Thromboembolism of the venous system (A) – used with Mayfield head holder device (D).	4. "nurik" (D) – similar letters.
5. A nerve for direct continuation of the posterior cord of brachial plexus.	5. Similar letters – muscle supplied by long thoracic nerve (A) (O).
6. One of the peripheral nerve injury classification systems (D).	6. 1/2 "chloro" (D) - muscle supplied by thoracodorsal nerve (A) - test for bleeding tendency (D).
7. A bone in the forearm – related to adrenal gland (A).	7. The first muscle located behind the medial malleolus (A) - one of the X-ray views with the X-ray tube angled 45 degrees down (D).
8. A muscle located in the posterior abdominal wall lateral to the psoas major muscle and superior to the iliacus muscle (A) – classification system for the severity of ulnar nerve injury (D).	8. Normal clinical sign denotes an intact anterior interosseous nerve – found in "stent".
9. A clinical test for carpal tunnel syndrome (D).	9. Poly-methyl-meth-acrylate bone cement (A) – runs inside.
10. Palsy of upper brachial plexus injury (C5,6) with the characteristic Bellhop's tip position of the hand.	10. Reduced by the use of tourniquet during peripheral nerve surgery (O).

A: Abbreviated. D: Distributed. O: Opposite

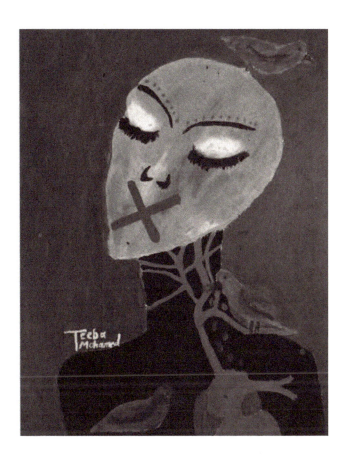

> "Silence is the real crime
> against humanity ..."

Nadezhda Mandelstam

9. Neurological examinations

	1	2	3	4	5	6	7	8	9	10
1										
2		■		■		■		■		
3										■
4						■				■
5										■
6						■				
7					■	■				
8			■							
9	■			■			■			
10			■							

Horizontal	Vertical
1. Type of pupil abnormalities also known as "tonic" pupil.	1. A sign considered as the upper limb equivalent of the Babinski sign.
2. Muscle in the leg supplied by tibial nerve (A) (O).	2. Found in" testosterone".
3. Gait abnormality seen in Parkinson's disease.	3. Alternative name for the Straight Leg Raise test. A Pioneer of pediatric neurosurgery who performed the first twin surgery - Type of brain hemorrhage (D).
4. Synonym of "Pseudo" (D)- ¾ of flap.	
5. A syndrome of Agraphia, Alexia, acalculia and neglect (D).	
6. The name of a grading system for TB meningitis (D) – 2/3 of "plexus" (O).	4. A type of meningeal cysts commonly found at the dorsal nerve root of the sacrum.
7. Should be examined in the limbs before the power (D)- 2/3 of "Saline" (O).	5. Supplied by T4 dermatome (D)- suffix indicates a tumor (O).
8. Similar letters- type of CSF shunts (A)- territory.	6. A target for deep brain stimulation in Parkinson's disease- similar letters.
9. Muscle in the leg supplied by peroneal nerve (A)- similar letters- Cognitive Functioning Scale (10-level scale) used to rate how people with brain injury are recovering and help to decide when a patient is ready for rehabilitation (O).	7. A partial or complete inability to read.
	8. A catecholamine that can be secreted by paraganglioma and causes life-threatening hypertension cardiac arrhythmias (D).
	9. A deep tendon reflex, mediated by the spinal nerves L2, L3, and L4 (D).
10. Used for clarification- a sign that describes the loss of postural control in darkness in patients with severely compromised proprioception.	10. Similar letters- a reflex that is one of the frontal release signs (O).

A: Abbreviated. D: Distributed. O: Opposite

10. History of neurosurgery

	1	2	3	4	5	6	7	8	9	10
1										
2										
3										
4										
5										
6										
7										
8										
9										
10										

Horizontal	Vertical
1. The founder of micro-neurosurgery.	1. Famous British neurosurgeon considered the first neurosurgeon in the world appointed to a hospital as "brain surgeon" (O) – similar letters.
2. An approach for resection of pituitary adenoma using endoscope (A) - 4/5 of "An Eye".	
3. Found in "Lyrica" – "sleepy" (D).	2. First name of the "Father of modern neurosurgery" (D) – *Japanese encephalitis* virus (A) (D).
4. Radial nerve superficial branch (A) – middle name of Portuguese neurologist gets the Nobel Prize 1949 (D).	
5. The father of microsurgical neuroanatomy – found in "stokes".	3. Pioneer of pediatric neurosurgery perform the first twin surgery – ½ "Chiari".
6. Type of stent-retriever used for mechanical thrombectomy (D) – 2/3 of "Henley" (O).	4. Found in "ETT" – 1/2 "culmen" (O).
7. First name of the developer of minimally invasive maxillary artery high-flow brain bypass surgery (D).	5. Inventor of x-ray (D).
	6. The great cerebral vein named after him (D) – orifice or opening (O).
8. Slovinian neurosurgeon pioneering the surgery of the cavernous sinus (D) - similar letters.	7. First name of neurosurgeon introduce the cisternostomy for severe traumatic brain injury – pioneer neurosurgeon (D).
9. First name of finish neurosurgeon develops the standard lateral supraorbital approach (D) – one of the parameters related to spino-pelvic alignment (O).	8. Founder of stereotactic radiosurgery (D).
	9. The inventor of cerebral angiography and frontal leucotomy (D).
10. Famous historical surgeon writes the "Canon of medicine", named the "vermis" and describe the spine biomechanics.	10. The inventor of cerebral bypass surgery using cardiac arrest (D).

A: Abbreviated. D: Distributed. O: Opposite

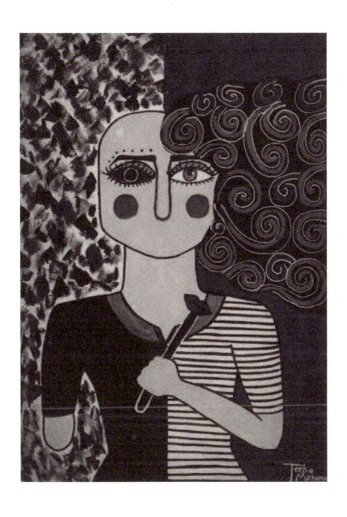

There is no perfect life
existed and there is no
perfect portrait completed!

perfection is the end point.

Section One: Answers

Basic Level Neurosurgery
Crossword Puzzles

Puzzles 1-40

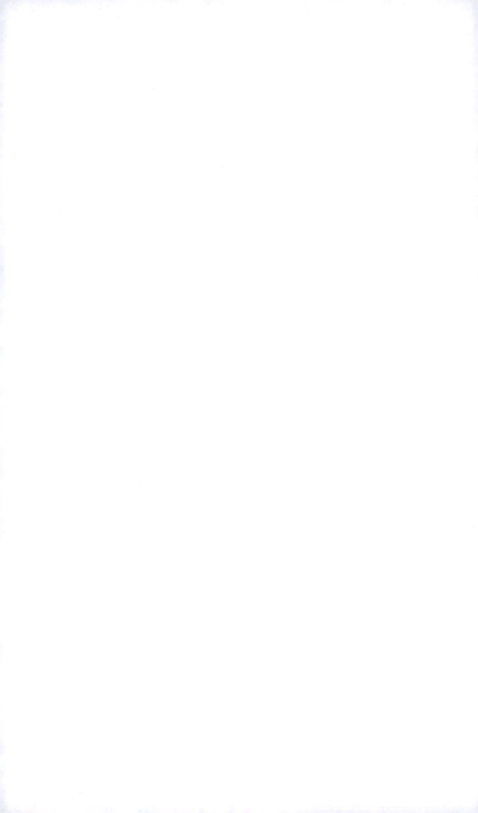

1. Facial Nerve Branches

									¹B			
									U			
									C			
									C			
		²C	E	R	V	I	C	A	L			
		H						L				
³Z	Y	G	O	M	A	T	I	C				
		R										
		D										
		⁴A	U	R	I	C	U	L	A	R		
		T										
		Y										
		⁵M	A	N	D	I	B	U	L	A	R	
		P										
⁶S	T	A	P	E	D	I	A	L				
		N										
	⁷D	I	G	A	S	⁸T	R	I	C			
						E						
						M						
						P						
						O						
						R						
						A						
						L						

2. Areas without Blood Brain Barrier

					¹S													
				²T	U	B	E	R	C	I	N	E	R	E	U	M		
					B													
					F													
				³O	R	G	A	N	U	M	V	A	S	C	U	L	O	S	U	M
					R													
				⁴N	E	U	R	O	H	Y	P	O	P	H	Y	S	I	S
					I													
					C													
			⁵P		A													
⁶C	H	O	R	O	I	D	P	L	E	X	U	S						
			N		O													
			E	⁷P	R	E	O	P	T	I	C	R	E	C	E	S	S
			A		G													
			L	⁸A	R	E	A	P	O	S	T	R	E	M	A			
			G		N													
			L															
			A															
			N															
			D															

3. Intracranial Aneurysms

```
M I D D L E C E R E B R A L
    I
    S U P E R I O R H Y P O P H Y S E A L
    T
    A N T E R I O R C O M M U N I C A T I N G
    L
    A
  I N T E R N A L C A R O T I D
    T
    E
  T R A U M A T I C
    I
  P O S T E R I O R C O M M U N I C A T I N G
    R
M Y C O T I C
    E
    R
    E
  B A S I L A R T I P
    R
O P H T H A L M I C
    L
```

4. Subarachnoid cisterns

```
. . . . . . . . . . . . . . M . . . . .
. . . . . . . . . . . . . . A . . . . .
. . . . . . . . . . . . . . G . . . . .
. . . . . L . . . . . . . . N . . . . .
. . . Q U A D R I G E M I N A L . . . C
. . . . . M . . . . . . . . . . . . . A
. . . . . I N T E R P E D U N C U L A R
. . . . . N . . . . . . . . . . . . . O
. . . . . A M B I E N T . . . . . . . T
. . . . . T . . . . . . . . . . . . . I
. . . . . E . . . . . . . . . . . . . D
. . . . . R . . . . . . . . . . . . . .
. . . . . M . . . . . . . . . . . . . .
. . . . . I . . . . . . . . . . . . . .
P R E P O N T I N E . . . . . . . . . .
. . . . . A . . . . . . . . . . . . . .
. . . S Y L V I A N . . . . . . . . . .
. . . . . I . . . . . . . . . . . . . .
. . . . . S U P R A S E L L A R . . . .
```

Cell labels: 1 M (down), 2 L (down), 3 Q (across), 4 C (down), 5 I (across), 6 A (across), 7 P (across), 8 S (across), 9 S (across)

5. Internal Carotid Artery branches:

¹P																
O																
²S	U	P	E	R	I	O	R	H	Y	P	O	P	H	Y	S	E	A	L
T																
E																
R																
I																
³O	P	H	T	H	A	L	M	I	C							
R																
C																
O																
⁴M	I	D	D	L	E	C	E	R	E	B	R	A	L			
M																
U																
⁵A	N	T	E	R	I	O	R	C	E	R	E	B	R	A	L	
I																
C																
⁶A	N	T	E	R	I	O	R	C	H	O	R	O	I	D	A	L
T																
I																
N																
G																

6. External Carotid Artery Branches

The crossword puzzle grid contains the following answers:

Across:
- 3. SUPERFICIALTEMPORAL
- 4. SUPERIORTHYROID
- 5. INTERNALMAXILLARY
- 6. POSTERIORAURICULAR
- 7. OCCIPITAL
- 8. LINGUAL

Down:
- 1. ASCENDINGPHARYNGEA
- 2. FACIAL

7. Carotid-vertebrobasilar Anastomoses

			¹H								
			Y								
			²P	R	O	A	T	L	A	N	T	A	L
			O								
³T	R	I	G	E	M	I	N	A	L		
			L								
			⁴O	T	I	C					
			S								
			S								
			A								
			L								

8. Cerebral veins

	S	U	P	E	R	I	O	R	P	E	T	R	O	S	A	L			
			R																
		D	E	E	P	M	I	D	D	L	E	C	E	R	E	B	R	A	L
			C																
			E																
		I	N	T	E	R	N	A	L	C	E	R	E	B	R	A	L		
			T																
			R																
	T	H	A	L	A	M	O	S	T	R	I	A	T	E					
			L																
			C																
			E																
		G	R	E	A	T	C	E	R	E	B	R	A	L					
			E																
	L	A	B	B	E														
			E																
T	R	O	L	A	R	D													
			L																
			A																
		R	O	S	E	N	T	H	A	L									

9. Aphasias

¹T	R	A	N	S	C	O	R	T	I	C	A	L	M	O	T	O	R
R															
A															
²N	O	M	I	N	A	L									
S															
³C	O	N	D	U	C	T	I	V	E						
O															
⁴B	R	O	C	A											
T															
I															
C															
A															
⁵G	L	O	B	A	L										
S															
⁶W	E	R	N	I	C	K	E								
N															
S															
O															
R															
Y															

10. Craniometric points

															¹E
															U
						²O	B	E	L	I	O	N			R
						P									I
						I			³B						O
						⁴S	T	E	F	A	N	⁵I	O	N
						T			S		N			
						H			I		I			
	⁶A	S	T	E	R	I	O	N		O		O		
						O			N		N			
⁷P	T	E	R	I	O	N								

11. Insertion points for ventriculo-peritoneal shunt:

		¹K								
		O								
		C								
		H								
		E			²K					
	³F	R	A	Z	I	E	R			
					E					
				⁴D	A	N	D	Y		

12. The age of intracerebral hemorrhage based on MR imaging.

¹H	Y	P	²E	R	A	C	U	T	E				
			A										
			R										
			³L	A	T	E	S	U	B	A	C	U	T	E
			Y										
			S										
	⁴A	C	U	T	E								
			B										
			A										
			⁵C	H	R	O	N	I	C				
			U										
			T										
			E										

13. Cranial foramina

				¹S	P	I	N	O	S	U	M	
				T								
			²H	Y	P	O	G	L	O	S	S	A	³L
				L								A
			⁴R	O	T	U	N	D	U	M		C
				M								E
⁵J	U	G	U	L	A	R						R
				S								U
				T								M
			⁶O	V	A	L	E					
				I								
				D								

14. Arteries supplying the internal capsule

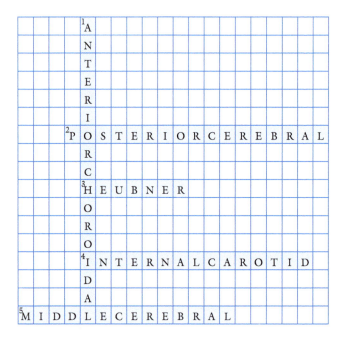

15. Brain Herniation syndromes

		¹S						
		²U	P	W	A	R	D	
		B						
		F						
³U	N	C	A	L				
		L						
		⁴C	E	N	T	R	A	L
		I						
	⁵T	O	N	S	I	L	L	A	R
		E						

16. Differential diagnoses of intraparenchymal Ring enhancing lesion

		¹M	E	T	A	S	T	A	S	I	S		
		U											
		L											
		²T	O	X	O	P	L	A	S	M	O	S	I	S
		I											
		P											
	³G	L	I	O	B	L	A	S	T	O	M	A	
		E											
⁴A	B	S	C	E	S	S						
		C											
		⁵L	Y	M	P	H	O	M	A				
		E											
		R											
		O											
		S											
		I											
		S											

17. Approaches for Selective Amygdalo-Hippocampectomy

¹S	U	B	T	E	M	P	O	R	A	L		
U												
P												
²T	R	A	N	S	S	Y	L	V	I	A	N	
A												
C												
E												
³T	R	A	N	S	S	U	L	C	A	L		
E												
B												
E												
L												
L												
A												
R												
⁴T	R	A	N	S	C	I	S	T	E	R	N	A	L
R												
A												
N												
S												
⁵T	R	A	N	S	T	E	M	P	O	R	A	L
E												
N												

18. Types of lumbar interbody fusion

					^{1}T
					L
			^{2}A		I
		^{3}O	L	I	F
	^{4}L		I		
^{5}P	L	I	F		
	I				
	F				

19. Types of Craniosynostosis

```
                    ¹T
                   ²B R A C H Y C E P H A L Y
                    I
                    G
                    O
                    N
                    O
                   ³S C A P H O C E P H A L Y
                    E
                   ⁴P L A G I O C E P H A L Y
                    H
⁵T U R R I C E P H A L Y
                    L
                    Y
```

20. Phacomatosis

¹N																
E																
U																
R																
²V	O	N	R	E	C	K	L	I	N	G	H	A	U	S	E	N
F																
I																
B																
R																
³V	O	N	H	I	P	P	E	L	L	I	N	D	A	U		
M																
A																
⁴T	U	B	E	R	O	U	S	S	C	L	E	R	O	S	I	S
O																
⁵S	T	U	R	G	E	W	E	B	E	R						
I																
S																

21. Pineal region tumors

	¹G	²E	R	M	I	N	O	M	A					
		M												
		B												
³T	E	R	A	T	O	M	A							
		Y												
		O												
⁴P	I	N	E	O	C	Y	T	O	M	A				
		A												
		L												
		⁵C	H	O	R	I	O	C	A	R	C	I	N	O	M	A
		A												
		R												
		C												
⁶P	I	N	E	O	B	L	A	S	T	O	M	A		
		N												
		O												
		M												
		A												

22. Peripheral nerves

				¹S	²C	I	A	T	I	C		
					O							
					³M	E	D	I	A	N		
					M							
					O							
			⁴U	L	N	A	R					
					P							
					E							
					⁵R	A	D	I	A	L		
					O							
					N							
					E							
					⁶A	X	I	L	L	A	R	Y
⁷T	I	B	I	A	L							

23. Types of Meningioma according to the location

		¹I											
		N											
		T											
	²F	O	R	A	M	E	N	M	A	G	N	U	M
		A											
		V											
³S	P	H	E	N	O	I	D	W	I	N	G		
		N											
		T											
	⁴P	A	R	A	S	A	G	I	T	T	A	L	
		I											
		C											
		U	⁵F										
	⁶O	L	F	A	C	T	O	R	Y	G	R	O	O	V	E
		A	L										
		R	X										

24. Histopathological types of Meningioma:

		¹M											
		E											
		N											
²P	A	P	I	L	L	A	R	Y					
		N											
		G											
		O											
		³T	R	A	N	S	I	T	I	O	N	A	L
		H											
		E											
		L		⁴C									
		I		H									
	⁵P	S	A	M	M	O	M	A	T	O	U	S	
		L		R									
				D									
				O									
				I									
				D									

25. Cerebral Metastasis

								¹R			
²C	O	³L	O	N				E			
		Y						N			
		⁴M	E	L	A	N	O	M	A		
		P						⁵L	U	N	G
	⁶T	H	Y	R	O	I	D				
		O									
		M									
⁷B	R	E	A	S	T						

26. jugular foramen syndromes

				¹T			
				A			
				P			
²S	³C	H	M	I	D	T	
	O			A			
	L						
	L						
⁴V	E	R	N	E	T		
	T						
	S						
⁵V	I	L	L	A	R	E	T
	C						
⁶J	A	C	K	S	O	N	
	R						
	D						

27. CSF shunt complications

1	2	3	4	5	6	7	8	9	10	11	12	13	14	15
		[1]A												
		S												
		C												
		I												
		T		[2]D										
	[3]P	E	R	I	T	O	N	I	T	I	[4]S			
[5]H		S		S							D		[6]S	
E				C							H		E	
[7]M	A	L	P	O	S	I	T	I	O	N			E	
O				N									D	
R				N									I	
R			[8]P	E	R	F	O	R	A	T	I	O	N	
H				C									G	
A				T										
G				I		[9]P								
E				[10]O	B	S	T	R	[11]U	C	T	[12]I	O	N
				N		E			L			N		
						U			C			F		
						D			E			E		
						O			R			C		
						C			A			T		
						Y			T			I		
						S			I			O		
						T			O			N		
									N					

28. Occipito-cervical junction ligaments

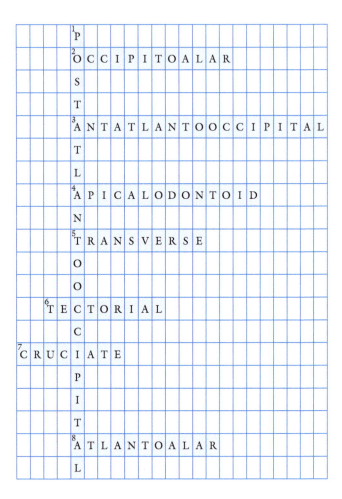

29. brainstem infarction syndromes

					¹W						
					E						
					B						
					E						
				²M	A	R	I	E	F	O	I	X
				I							
				³L	O	C	K	E	D	I	N	
				L							
			⁴W	A	L	L	E	N	B	E	R	G
				R							
				⁵D	E	J	E	R	I	N	E	
				G							
				U							
				⁶B	E	N	E	D	I	K	T	
				L							
⁷C	L	A	U	D	E						
				⁸R	E	I	N	H	O	L	D	

30. Spinal cord syndromes

					¹C	A	U	D	A	E	Q	U	I	N	A
					O										
			²C	E	N	T	R	A	L						
					U										
					S										
					³M	Y	E	L	O	P	A	T	H	Y	
					E										
					⁴D	O	R	S	A	L					
					U										
⁵V	E	N	T	R	A	L									
					L										
					A										
			⁶B	R	O	W	N	S	E	Q	U	A	R	D	
					I										
					S										

31. Nerve supply

				¹T	I	B	I	²A	L			³P			
								X				U		⁴R	
				⁵M	E	D	I	A	N			D		A		⁶F
								L				E		D		E
				⁷M				L				N		I		M
				U				A				D		A		O
				⁸S	U	P	R	A	S	C	A	P	U	L	A	R
⁹P	H	R	E	N	I	C		Y				L				A
				U									¹⁰P			L
				¹¹L	O	N	G	T	H	O	R	¹²A	C	I	C
				O								I		N	
		¹³A	C	C	E	S	S	O	R	Y		N			
				U										¹⁴U
				¹⁵T	H	O	R	A	C	O	D	O	R	S	A	L
				A											N
¹⁶I	N	F	E	R	I	N	R	G	L	U	T	E	A	L		A
				E											R
				¹⁷O	B	T	U	R	A	T	O	R			
				U										
				¹⁸S	U	B	¹⁹S	C	A	P	U	L	A	R
							C							
							I							
							A							
							T							
							I							
							C							

32. Cerebral sulci

The completed crossword grid reads as follows:

- 1 Down: LATERALL
- 2 Down: CALLL
- 3/4 Across: PARIETOOCCIPITAL
- 4 Down: ANTERER
- 5 Across: CENTRAL
- 6 Across: INFERIORFRONTAL
- 7 Across: PRECENTRAL
- 8 Across: SUPERIORTEMPORAL
- 9 Across: CINGULATE
- 10 Across: INTRAPARIETAL
- 11 Across: MARGINAL
- 12 Across: CALCARINE
- 13 Across: POSTCENTRAL

												L	
				C								A	
				A								T	
				L								E	
				L								R	
	P	A	R	I	E	T	O	O	C	C	I	P	I	T	A	L
		N		S								L	
C	E	N	T	R	A	L		A					
		E						L					
		R											
		I	N	F	E	R	I	O	R	F	R	O	N	T	A	L
		O											
	P	R	E	C	E	N	T	R	A	L			
		A											
		S	U	P	E	R	I	O	R	T	E	M	P	O	R	A	L
		C											
		E											
	C	I	N	G	U	L	A	T	E				
		D											
		I	N	T	R	A	P	A	R	I	E	T	A	L
		N											
M	A	R	G	I	N	A	L						
		G											
	C	A	L	C	A	R	I	N	E				
		M											
		U											
P	O	S	T	C	E	N	T	R	A	L			

33. Cerebral gyri - surface anatomy

Across / Down answers filled in the crossword grid:

- 1 (down): ANGULAR
- 2 (across): SUPERIORTEMPORAL
- 2 (down): SUPPLEMENTARY
- 3 (across): PARSTRIANGULAR
- 4 (across): PRECENTRAL
- 5 (across): PRECUNEUS
- 6 (across): FRONTALEYEFIELD
- 7 (down): LINGUAL
- 8 (across): POSTCENTRAL
- 9 (down): HESCHL
- 10 (across): SUPRAMARGINAL

34. Pupil abnormalities

					¹A	N	I	S	O	C	O	R	I	A	
²H	O	R	N	E	R										
					G										
					Y										
					L										
					L										
					R										
				³H	O	L	M	E	S	A	D	I	E		
					B										
					E										
			⁴M	A	R	C	U	S	G	U	N	N			
					T										
					S										
					O										
				⁵N	O	N	R	E	A	C	T	I	V	E	

35. Peripheral nerve palsy syndromes

¹P	I	R	I	F	O	R	²M	I	S								
							E										
					³C	A	R	P	A	L	T	U	N	N	E	L	
							A										
			⁴G	U	I	L	L	A	I	N	B	A	R	R	E		
							G										
				⁵C	U	B	I	T	A	L	T	U	N	N	E	L	
							A										
							P										
				⁶S	A	T	U	R	D	A	Y	N	I	G	H	T	
							R										
							E										
				⁷S	T	R	A	W	B	E	R	R	Y	P	I	C	K	E	R
							T										
							H										
							E						⁸G				
				⁹C	A	P	T	A	I	N	C	H	A	I	R		
							I						U				
				¹⁰C	H	A	R	C	O	¹¹T	M	A	R	I	¹²E	T	O	O	¹³T	H
							A			A			R		N		A
							R			S			B		S		R
							S						S		C		D
							A								A		Y
							L								N		
							T								A		
							U								L		
							N										
							N										
							E										
							L										

36. The Orbit

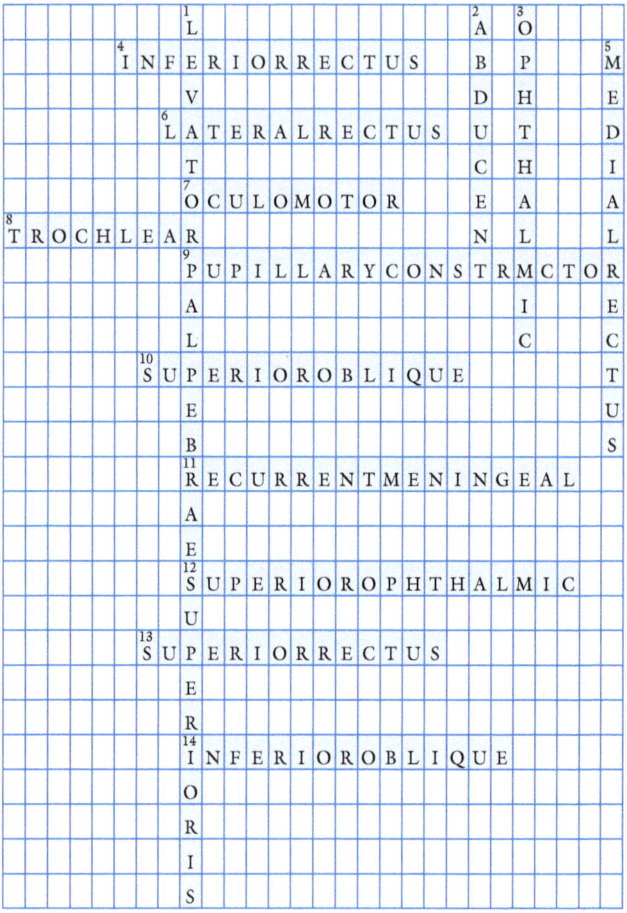
1 LEVATORPALPEBRAESUPERIORIS
2 ABDUCENT
3 OPHTHALMIC
4 INFERIORRECTUS
5 MEDIALRECTUS
6 LATERALRECTUS
7 OCULOMOTOR
8 TROCHLEAR
9 PUPILLARYCONSTRMCTOR
10 SUPERIOROBLIQUE
11 RECURRENTMENINGEAL
12 SUPERIOROPHTHALMIC
13 SUPERIORRECTUS
14 INFERIOROBLIQUE

37. Spinal cord tracts

```
   P
D  O  R  S  A  L  C  O  L  U  M  N
   S
   T
V  E  S  T  I  B  U  L  O  S  P  I  N  A  L
   R
   I
   O
   R  E  T  I  C  U  L  O  S  P  I  N  A  L
   S
S  P  I  N  O  T  E  C  T  A  L
   I
A  N  T  E  R  I  O  R  S  P  I  N  O  T  H  A  L  A  M  I  C
   O
   C  O  R  T  I  C  O  S  P  I  N  A  L
   E
   R  U  B  R  O  S  P  I  N  A  L
   E
   B
   E
   L  A  T  E  R  A  L  S  P  I  N  O  T  H  A  L  A  M  I  C
   L
   A  N  T  E  R  I  O  R  S  P  I  N  O  C  E  R  E  B  E  L  L  A  R
   R
```

38. Magnetic Resonance Spectroscopy (MRS)

	¹C	H	O	L	I	N	E
	R						
	E						
²L	A	C	T	A	T	E	
	T						
	I						
	³N	A	A				
	E						

39. Complications of Subthalamic Nucleus (STN) Deep Brain Stimulation (DBS).

	¹A										
²I	N	F	E	R	O	M	E	D	I	A	L
	T										
³M	E	D	I	A	L						
	R										
⁴P	O	S	T	E	R	I	O	R			
	L										
	⁵A	N	T	E	R	I	O	R			
	T										
	E										
	R										
	A										
	⁶L	A	T	E	R	A	L				

40. Dermatomal levels

```
                                               T
                                             F   H
                                             O  F I R S T L U M B A R
                                             U   R
                                             R   D
                                             T   C
                                             H   E
                                             L   R
                                             U   V
                                             M  F I R S T S A C R A L
                                             B   C
                   S                         A   A
                   E I G H T H C E R V I C A L
                   V
                 S E C O N D C E R V I C A L
                   N
             S I X T H C E R V I C A L
                   H
 T E N T H T H O R A C I C
                   E
             F O U R T H T H O R A C I C
         F         V
         I     F I F T H C E R V I C A L
         F         C
     S I X T H T H O R A C I C
     E   H   H       L
     C   L   I
     O   U   R
     N   M   D
     D   B   L
     S   A   U
     A   R   M
     C       B
     R       A
     A       R
     L
```

Answer key

Down
- 1. THIRD CERVICAL
- 2. FOURTH LUMBAR
- 5. SEVENTH CERVICAL
- 11. FIFTH LUMBAR
- 13. SECOND SACRAL
- 14. THIRD LUMBAR

Across
- 3. FIRST LUMBAR
- 4. FIRST SACRAL
- 6. EIGHTH CERVICAL
- 7. SECOND CERVICAL
- 8. SIXTH CERVICAL
- 9. TENTH THORACIC
- 10. FOURTH THORACIC
- 12. FIFTH CERVICAL
- 13. SIXTH THORACIC

Section Two: Answers

Advanced Level Neurosurgery Crossword Puzzles

1. Pediatric neurosurgery

	1	2	3	4	5	6	7	8	9	10
1	S	I	N	C	I	P	I	T	A	L
2	I	N	F	E	C	T	I	O	N	
3	S	F		A	A		H	R	A	I
4	O	E	T				G			
5	T	R	T			E	L	O	M	
6	S	I	T	I	G	N	I	N	E	M
7	O	O		A	H	E	S	I	T	T
8	N	R	O	H		G	N		H	T
9	Y		P	T	T		O	X	Y	
10	S	Y	N	D	A	C	T	Y	L	Y

2. Vascular neurosurgery (1)

	1	2	3	4	5	6	7	8	9	10
1	D	A	V	F	I	S	T	U	L	a
2	U	R	A		S	T	A	N	E	c
3	R	U	M			a	R	I	U	M
4	A	B	r	N	T		B			A
5	L	A	n	I	P	s		d	v	T
6	R		s	L	A		s	I	R	S
7	I	M	o	S		S	A	R		
8	N	I	e	v		A	C	B	N	
9	G		A	Y	O	M	a	Y	o	M
10	S	U	c	a		E		H	I	V

3. Vascular neurosurgery (2)

	1	2	3	4	5	6	7	8	9	10
1	A	N	E	U	R	Y	S	M		M
2	N	A	G	V	E	S	I	E	A	T
3	G	V	A		C	P	L		L	O
4	I	I	H		U	E	A		U	R
5	O	G	R		R	L	R		T	
6	M	A	R		R	I	O	P	S	T
7	A	T	O	O	E	P	P	R	I	N
8		I	M		N	E	M		F	
9	M	O	E		T		E		C	S
10	I	N	H			I	T	U	C	S

4. Neuro-oncology

	1	2	3	4	5	6	7	8	9	10
1	A	C	E	T	A	T	S	O	R	P
2	M	A	D		M		T	R	T	A
3	O	L	I	V	E				O	P
4	I	C	A	A		F	R		M	I
5	G	I	T				D	O	A	L
6	N	F			O	B	M	O	E	L
7	I	I			L	R	I	Y	T	A
8	N	E		D	I	O	D	B	A	R
9	E	D	A	R	G	W	O	L		Y
10	M		A	M	O	N	E	D	A	

5. Functional neurosurgery

	1	2	3	4	5	6	7	8	9	10
1	D	E	P	R	E	S	S	I	O	N
2	I	P	L	Y	E	P	S	E		O
3	R	I	A	S	G	A	E	G	L	S
4	E	P	G			S	P	U	A	N
5	C		I	T	N	T		D	T	I
6	T	M	O	N	A	I	S		C	K
7		U		W	S	C		Z	E	R
8	S	B	D		C	I	T	O	R	A
9	T	E	G	R	E	T	O	L		P
10	N	S		H	T	Y	R	E		

6. Neurotrauma

	1	2	3	4	5	6	7	8	9	10
1	C	O	N	C	U	S	S	I	O	N
2	A	R	E	I	O	S	O	S	U	N
3	R	E	W	O	P		G	A	T	
4	E	S		R		P		U	L	T
5	E	P	I	D	U	R	A	L		A
6	N	A	C	S	T	C	K	C	E	N
7	I	T	D		E		L	L	I	G
8	N	I	A	R	B	D	I	M		E
9	G	N	O	P	G	N	I	P		N
10		O	N	C		I	N	L	E	T

7. Spine

	1	2	3	4	5	6	7	8	9	10
1	F	L	A	V	U	M		B	T	P
2	I	O	N	R		L	E	T	A	r
3	L	A	S	E	G	U	E		W	
4	O	D	M	I	C		E	L	A	k
5			B	B	O	C		O	N	y
6	A	F	S		S	o	C	L	A	P
7	C	A	R	N	L	E	T		R	H
8	D	R	I	H	T		A	A		O
9	F	E	L	P		G	R	A	S	S
10		b	U	R	S	I	T	I	S	

8. Peripheral nerves

	1	2	3	4	5	6	7	8	9	10
1	N	E	U	R	E	C	T	O	M	Y
2	I		K	U	E	L	P	K	M	
3	A	P	L	N	E	H		S	A	G
4	V	T		K				I	P	N
5	R	A	D	I	A	L		G		I
6	E		T		S	D	O	N	E	D
7	U	L	N	A			T		N	E
8	Q	L		A	T	R	W	S	T	E
9	E		T			I	N	T	E	L
10	D	U	C	H	E	N	E	E	R	B

9. Neurological examination:

	1	2	3	4	5	6	7	8	9	10
1	H	O	L	M	E	S	A	D	I	E
2	O		A		P	T		I		E
3	F	E	S	T	I	N	A	N	T	
4	F	S	E	A	L		L	A	P	
5	M	T	G	R	N	S	E	N	A	
6	A	R	U	L	P		X	E	L	p
7	N	T	E	O			I	L	A	S
8	N	N		V	A		A	R	E	A
9		E	D		M	M		A	L	R
10	I	E		R	O	M	B	E	R	G

10. History of neurosurgery

	1	2	3	4	5	6	7	8	9	10
1	Y	A	S	A	R	G	I	L		
2	E	E	A		N	E	Y	E		L
3	L	Y	C		E	L	P	E	Y	S
4	S	R	N		G	A	E	S		R
5	R	H	O	T	O	N		K	O	T
6	O	V	R	E	T		Y	L	N	E
7	H				E	S	A	L	M	E
8		E	C	L	N	O	D		Z	Z
9	A	J	H	U		A	D		I	P
10	A	V	I	C	E	N	N	A		

References:

- The Handbook of Neurosurgery
- www.Radiopedia.com
- www.upsurgeon.com
- The American Association of Neurosurgery website
- www.Google.com

Thanks for your time